A Natural Solution

To

Health and Healing

Linda Ybarra N.D., Ph.D.

Certified Holistic Health Practitioner

No part of this publication may be reproduced, stored in a retrieval system or transmitted in any way by any means, electronic, mechanical, photocopy, recording or otherwise without the prior permission of the author except as provided by USA copyright law..

Published in the United States of America

ISBN: -13:978-1495205231

Dedication Page

I dedicate this book to all those willing
to take part in their own health and
healing.

Table of Contents

Introduction

What I have to share can improve your life.

That is my reason for writing this book.

Health is a mind, body, spirit connection that you can improve, obtain, and maintain over time. The **little** choices you make every day are the contributing factors to good health or *dis-ease.*

When we bombarded our body with toxic ingredients and chemicals from our personal care products, the food we eat, or just going through our daily lives, the body can hit toxic overload. These accumulated toxins attack the body's immune system causing disease. Learning to avoid and **eliminate** the amount of toxins we ingest or come into contact with will improve the risk we run of getting sick.

Healthy choices compound over time as do the unhealthy choices. You are literally building your health one day at a time. Just like a bank account that you add to or deplete. You can improve your health like you improve your wealth, a little bit every day.

It is my hope to give you some easy, fun, inexpensive and simple **but oh-so-powerful** choices for a vital and energetic life.

I will start with my story. It is proof that good health is obtainable at any age and improving health can start at any time. Best of all it does not require an over-structured, tiring regiment to follow. In fact, taking the stress out of having to live by unrealistic guidelines or trying every 'new miracle product' is freeing! This process can even be fun! Especially when you include therapies like: laughter, color and music in your healthy lifestyle choices.

XXXX

~ *Linda*

XXXX

My Story

I am the mother of two beautiful grown daughters. My girls were two and four years old when I found myself trying to find a job while the details of my divorce settlement were being hashed- out. Not a situation I wanted for my girls or myself, mostly because I come from a family of divorce.

I made a decision that I would make this divorce as civil as I could in order to keep the girls' father, and his family, as involved in my girls' lives as possible. Through my experiences, I learned what I wanted to do differently. Also, I had high expectations for how actively involved I wanted to stay in my girls' daily life. I committed to the girls being my first priority and I did my best to see that through.

The years took their toll on my health. By the time my girls graduated from high school, my overall physical health had deteriorated. My list of health issues mounted until I was no longer able to work the various jobs that helped me support myself and my girls through the years.

In my search for answers and help, I went to an old-school, Chinese acupuncturist. It was important to me to find and use the acupuncture method that had been around and used successfully for thousands of years. I believe that newer is NOT always better! I wanted to experience the ancient, proven method of Chinese acupuncture. My visit with the acupuncturist is where I found out that all my organs were shutting down, causing the Chronic fatigue, and pain that I was experiencing.

The depression, pain, complete exhaustion and inability participate in the daily routine of life is the point at which I was ready to give up. I was ready to check out of this physical body.

That is when I moved to Sedona, Arizona. In hind-sight I recognize that I needed a gradual separation for myself and my girls. I wanted to know that they would be fine without me. But, when my girls became aware of the situation, they let me know that they were not going to accept my choice to give up.

So I **needed** to find a way to get well!

At that time, I had no health insurance and no faith in conventional medicine. I had worked for doctors in the past. I feel like conventional medicine is barbaric at times and more damaging than helpful in most instances. So, I wanted to try a natural path to health, even before I knew much about what that entailed

I started taking supplements. That was my first avenue for experimenting. I would go to a health food store and get what they would recommend for the most troubling symptoms at the time.

Unable to work forced me to seek disability benefits and during the process of qualifying for disability I discovered that I had degenerative arthritis of the spine (explaining the severe back pain) along with a multitude of other ailments.

Being on disability enabled me to apply for vocational rehabilitation, which allowed me the opportunity to study natural health ending up with a PhD, and N.D. I used my studies as a way to climb my way back, **ever so slowly**, to health.

Today I am healthy and feel better than I have in many years! I have more energy than I could possibly expect for my age. I have learned how to eat and live to maintain that health. I am now an active, vibrant, participating member of society. I no longer have arthritis of any kind and I feel better than I could have imagined all those years ago.

Now, I want to share what I have learned through experience and my studies with anyone that wants to apply these changes for their own good.

I incorporated natural remedies, natural health, prevention, and living green into simple, daily habits that improved my quality of life. My daughters have even refers to me as "The *MacGyver* of Natural Health." Along the way, I learned that living green brings us back to nature and helps the healing process as well as the environment. Everyone wins!

This is available and beneficial for anyone at any age!

Now that I have come so far and been so successful with my own health, I am hoping to share with others so they can do the same with their own health.

Every little healthy thing you do for your body is beneficial and accumulates over time, just as every harmful thing you do to your body does.

Incorporating some easy, healthy habits into your daily routine can mean the difference between health and *dis-ease*.

I want you to experience the sense of independence and comfort you get from being in control of your own health.

Prevention, maintenance, and natural healing remedies can help you get to this point. It is important that you see that simple, daily habits can make a huge impact on your current and future health!

This is a *process* and it allows for lee-way, liberties, and choices. **But** it is important to remember that too many bad choices result in too much toxic build up. That makes a major difference in the way you feel and your overall health!

Acknowledgements

I want to acknowledge my **Gina** and **Dana** for their unwavering love and support.

My mom for her help through some rough times.

My son-law for the wonderful lifestyle he provides for my daughter and grandkids.

And My **Antonio** and **Bella**: thank you for the **world's best hugs and kisses!**

Personal

Care

Dental Care

Holistic dentists perform dentistry that is good for the body, teeth, and gums. Holistic dentists believe that what goes into your mouth can affect your entire body and your overall health. Here are some questions to ask a dentist when searching for the right dentist for you:

1. Does the dentist use air and water abrasion instead of a drill?

2. Does the dentist do composite testing for compatibility?

3. Does the dentist use digital imaging instead of old fashion x-ray? (This technique uses nearly 85% less radiation)

4. Does the dentist have an ozone teeth cleaning machine?

5. Does the dentist have updated vacuum and mercury removal ventilation equipment and use the newest procedures?

Not all dentists that advertise as holistic really use the holistic approach. By asking these questions, you can find a natural, holistic dentist.

Why choose a holistic dentist?

Holistic dentist do **not** use mercury amalgam fillings.

Mercury is a Toxin and even a **very small amount**s is a health risk not worth taking. Think about this.....mercury stays in your mouth for years emitting trace amounts that leaches into your system on a daily basis. Every time you chew you stimulate an additional release of mercury vapors over and over again. That is just **not** healthy!

Oh, and did I mention that air and water abrasion require no filling (mercury amalgam) and no injection (the need for early detection comes into play here).

Your dentist should at least meet, if not surpass, guidelines for safe removal of mercury amalgam fillings.

Holistic dentists are generally against the use of fluoride. Research indicates excessive Fluoride can cause cancer and bone problems and there is no benefit to teeth from ingested fluoride.
Be sure to check labels when looking to purchase toothpaste and mouth.

Root canals **are not** recommended by holistic dentists because the chemicals used are toxic (one being formaldehyde). Formaldehyde is a known carcinogen that causes dizziness, headaches, fatigue, and immune dysfunction. Another reason to avoid a root canal is because of the bacteria left behind after the procedure that can lead to heart disease or breast cancer. Removing the infected tooth is a better choice.

Oral Hygiene Naturally

Holistic Dentistry provides natural cleaning techniques like ozone therapy.

A great way to keep gums and teeth healthy is to brush with aluminum-free baking soda. Use Aluminum free baking soda instead of toothpaste. A soft toothbrush is always preferred for gum health. Baking soda used instead of toothpaste will whiten teeth and leave them feeling cleans and smooth like a dentist cleaning without the dentist or the chemicals.

If you use toothpaste always check the labels and use a clean, natural toothpaste.

Another Natural oral hygiene tip is to use Food-grade hydrogen peroxide added to your natural toothpaste. Once or twice a week will help fight gum disease and whiten teeth. It is important to use **food-grade** hydrogen peroxide **only** and use it **sparingly,** a little goes a long way! One drop on your toothpaste will do the trick. Be careful to avoid direct contact with your skin.

Skin Care

It is important to make wise choices with the skin and hair care products you use. There are many ingredients and chemicals in these products that you want to avoid because they are easily absorbed through the pores causing health problems. The skin is the largest organ of the body. What goes on your skin is absorbed directly into the blood system. The average woman absorbs as much as 5 pounds of chemicals each year just from their personal care products.

.

Ingredients to *Avoid* in Personal Care Products

Ingredients to avoid in shampoo, lotions, and cosmetics; because what we use topically is absorbed internally: Read labels and choose carefully. Your health depends on it!

Methylparaben, Propylparaben, Butylparaben, and Ethylparaben: Even though these ingredients are cancer causing and toxic they are used to extend shelf life in most personal care products in the United States.

Parabens (Methyl, Propyl, Butyl, and Ethylparaben) are found in deodorants, antiperspirants, sunscreens, shampoos, and makeup of all kinds. Studies have reportedly found paraben concentrations, in women with breast tumors, at twice the average level. Please read labels to avoid products with parabens

Petrolatum: Petrolatum commonly known as petroleum jelly, is a byproduct of petroleum and is used in the manufacturing of personal care products. The side effects of petrolatum include suffocation of the skin, premature aging, aggravated acne and finding petrolatum byproducts in breast tumors.
Petrolatum and mineral oil promotes sun damage and tends to interfere with the body's own natural moisturizing mechanism but is found in many popular lip products.

Propylene Glycol: Over time, this additive can cause cancer, toxic reactions and allergies.

Imidazonlidinyl Urea and Diazolidinyl Urea: These chemicals are toxic, causing dermatitis and they release formaldehyde.

PVP/VA Copolymer: This is used in many hairsprays. Toxic polymers contribute to foreign bodies in the lungs.

Sodium Lauryl Sulfate: It causes hair loss, eye irritations, skin rashes, and scalp scurf similar to dandruff (used in shampoos and cosmetics)

Synthetic Colors: These additives are believed to be cancer-causing agents.

Stearalkonium Chloride: This compound is used in hair conditioners and creams. It was developed by the fabric industry as a fabric softener, but because it is cheaper and easier to use than proteins you find it in hair conditioning formulas.

Triethanolamine: This chemical is used in cosmetics and can be toxic if absorbed into the body over a long period of time. Triethanolamine causes allergic reactions including eye problems, dryness of hair, and skin.

Why Organic Deodorant?

The ingredients in many deodorant products could be harmful to your health. There is much speculation about the role of deodorants as a possible connection with breast cancer.

There is a strong possibility that aluminum in deodorants may contribute to Alzheimer's disease. Ingredients, such as aluminum, act like estrogen and can upset your hormonal balance.

You should always read the ingredients before you purchase a deodorant. It is critical to your health because *remember* what you put on your skin is absorbed directly into your bloodstream. Harmful ingredients in your blood have potentially harmful effects on your health.

Some ingredients to avoid when choosing your deodorant include: aluminum chlorohydrate, aluminum compounds, parabens (methyl, ethyl, propyl, benzyl and butyl, triclosan, talc (a carcinogen), and propylene glycol.

Banish Body Order!

If you want your deodorant to work more effectively, use a small dusting of aluminum-free baking soda on your underarms after applying your natural deodorant. Sweating is natures' way of detoxing but odor is offensive so give this natural solution a try.

Foods for Great Skin

A dull, dry complexion is a reflection of improper nutrition. With a better diet, you can change that.

Nutrition and good health is essential for preserving your skin's youthful look and for maintaining your skins' primary function of protecting your organs from outside elements. By implementing a few skin-protecting foods into your diet, you can have great looking healthy skin.

Here are some foods for great looking skin:

Avocados are abundant in essential oils and B-complex vitamins that nourish your skin, inside and out. Niacin is important for healthy skin, and avocados contain Niacin. Niacin is an anti-inflammatory and soothes irritated, red, and blotchy skin. A great avocado face-mask will solve dry skin problems instantly.

Mango. **M**angos' are a repairing food. The Vitamin A in a mango helps maintains and repairs skin cells, and fight free radical damage that can age the skin.

Almonds. Almonds are full of Vitamin E. Vitamin E moisturizes dry skin and its antioxidants protect against skin damage and aging.

Cottage Cheese. The selenium and vitamin E in cottage cheese make a powerful free-radical fighting antioxidant duo.

Acerola Cherries. This cherry fights skin damage and wrinkles. It also plays a central role in the production of collagen, the structural protein in your skin.

Baked Potatoes. A simple, white baked potato produces elastin. A protein, elastin is a connective tissue that allows tissues in the body to resume their shape after stretching or contracting. Elastin helps the skin return to its original suppleness after harmful environmental exposure, stretch marks, or drastic weight loss/gain.

Flaxseed Oil. This tiny grain is an Omega 3 powerhouse! By adding flaxseed to your morning cereal, or taking the oil as a vitamin supplement, flaxseed can help fight inflammation in the skin as well as helping prevent diabetes and cancer!

Eye Health

It is never too early or too late to reap benefits from natural eye care. I believe there are three main ways in which to do this.

Prevention

Nutrition

Exercise

Prevention

Avoid free radicals at all costs. This includes auto exhaust, and spray cans. Try to soak up early-morning and early-evening exposure to outdoor light for 10 to 15 minutes daily, without glasses.

Nutritional Eye Support

A healthier diet, including carrots, dark colored vegetables, and sweet potatoes all contain beta carotene. Spinach, apricots, winter squash, cantaloupe, broccoli, liver, and peaches are also full of vitamin A and beta carotene that promote eye health.

Herbs can also help. Eyebright, bilberry, and ginkgo biloba all contain vitamins that promote eye health.

Eye Exercises

Those of us that work under artificial lighting and in front of computer screens all day, need a little extra TLC for the eyes. If you wear glasses, make sure to do the following exercises without your glasses to lessen your dependence on them.

Start this exercise for your eyes by looking as far as possible to the left then right, then up and down holding for 8 seconds in each direction.

Do figure 8's with your eyes, and then make circles for about 20 seconds.

Focus on a pencil in front of your face, then pick out a point about 20 plus feet

away point to maintain focus. Force
eyes to relax, and then turn your focus
back to the pencil. Holding for eight
seconds at a time. This is especially
beneficial for computer users.

Pinhole viewing exercise is helping
people improve their vision without
laser surgery. The glasses have multiple
holes in both lenses and are most
effective when worn while watching TV
or reading. Pinholes are also great for
computer operators. Computer screens
exhaust and strain eyes quickly. These
glasses allow your eyes to relax.
Make sure you do not use pinhole
glasses when driving or doing any

activity where peripheral vision is required.

Let the Sun Shine In!

The Benefits of Sunshine.

Sunshine in moderation is a vital part of healthy living. Sunlight plays an important role in the recovery from chronic disease. Sunlight can be part of the curing process in almost every affliction.

We all know that the body produces vitamin D with exposure to the sun but I want to point out that sunshine exposure reduces the symptoms of depression through endorphin production. Sunshine increases circulation, strengthens the immune system, increases metabolism, helps maintain blood sugar levels, and we have talked about the benefits of a few minutes (five to fifteen minutes) of early morning or early evening exposure sunshine for the eyes. Sunshine also reduces the risk of Alzheimer's. So what's not to love about a moment in the sun? Be sure to consult with your dermatologist about the right sunscreen.

Nail Polish

Conventional nail polishes contain many toxic chemicals like formaldehyde, toluene, acetone, and dibutyl-phthalate that can cause health problems

Formaldehyde is a known carcinogen that causes dizziness, headaches, fatigue, and immune dysfunction

Toluene may affect the nervous system with symptoms such as: tiredness, confusion, weakness, memory loss, skin irritation and liver and heart damage. In high levels may affect the kidneys.

Phthalates affect hormone function. Studies have linked phthalates to early puberty in girls and low sperm count in men.

Acetone is a chemical used in nail polish, nail polish remover, and in many household products. Poisoning from acetone may occur from breathing in fumes or absorption through the skin or nails.

The best choice for beautiful nails is **buffing**. Buffing treatments can improve circulation in the nail bed, which can help to keep nails healthy, strong and improves nail growth. The process used to buff nails helps to make nails shinny without the need for additional products.

Dry Skin Brushing

Did you know that the skin is the largest organ in the body?

It is also responsible for one-fourth of the body's detoxification each day, eliminating up to two **pounds** of waste acids daily! It protects your organs from the elements! Skin also plays a key role in the immune system by keeping out potential infectious. And it transforms sunlight into vitamin D.

Your skin receives one third of all the blood that circulates in the body. When your blood is full of toxic materials, it reflectes as acne, dull aged and wrinkled skin and broken blood vessels. The skin is the last organ to receive nutrients in the body, yet the first to shows signs of imbalance or deficiency.

Dry skin brushing supports skin health
and requires very little time or money.

It only takes a few minutes every day.
All you need is a simple body brush
made with natural fiber bristles. A long
handle brush will make reaching the
entire area of your back much easier.
You can use a loofah or skin exfoliation
glove or even a towel if necessary. I
even use a soft dry brush for my face
each morning.
Use sweeping or circular strokes toward
the heart.
Be sure to clean your brushes with a
castile soap every week or so.

Benefits of dry skin brushing:

Reduce cellulite When you massage and invigorate the skin, it starts to break up the toxic deposits of stored fat tissues that cause cellulite. Try to be patient though; this is not an overnight quick fix. Daily brushing is required for several months to start to see results.

Cleanses the lymphatic system - The lymphatic system is your body's natural cleaning system. White blood cells transport nutrients and remove waste. If white blood cells do not move through the body quickly enough, can become swollen causing, inflammation. Inflammation is an attempt of the body to heal itself. Along with exercise, skin brushing can assist the lymphatic system's natural cleansing rhythm.

Strengths the immune system – Stimulating the lymphatic system helps the body to detoxify by moving waste-matter out faster. Removing toxins more rapidly through the system can lessen the duration of infections and illnesses.

Remove dead skin Dry skin brushing removes dead skin cells, opens the pores to enhance the skins ability to remove waste from the body, and improves movement of nutrients and oxygenated blood to the skin.

Tightens the skin Dry brushing rejuvenates nerve endings resulting in more toned muscles. **So** instead of spending money on creams and medical procedures, you can prevent premature aging by invigorating the nerve endings in the skin! Increasing blood flow to skin, as well as removing dead cells, helps create new, tighter skin, and overall skin health.

Tones the muscles - Stimulating nerve endings in the skin, will activate individual muscle fibers, resulting in toner muscles.

Increases Circulation Increased circulation and blood flow helps promote cell growth and organ function.

Your skin is better able to fight off bacteria and infections. Your heart rate lowers, heart muscles relax and your blood pressure evens out..

Dry Skin brushing is easy, inexpensive and invigorating!

Lotion

Moisturized Skin is Happy Skin!

Dry skin has a **decreased** capacity to heal. This makes skin far more susceptible to various forms of skin damage such as sun exposure.

Dry skin is also more prone to skin infections and irritants.

Most people over forty have some degree of skin dryness and need to moisturize. Skin dryness tends to be more prevalent in women near, during or after menopause.

Moisturizers are essential to skin care. Applying moisturizers regularly keep your skin hydrated, soft, supple, and young-looking. But choose wisely! Use organic, clean products. You can find some of my personal suggestions in *"my Favorite Things,"* section.

Medicinal Lotion

Lotion is not just for helping keep your skin soft and smooth. Lotions can actually heal your body from the outside, in!

A lotion that my family has used for years is a combination of Glucosamine, MSM, & Arnica lotion. It helps relieve pain, is an anti-inflammatory, helps prevent bruising and helps your body repair its self.

Glucosamine sulfate helps to keep joints in the body operating smoothly. Glucosamine sulfate is a simple molecular building block used to support mobility and flexibility in joints.

Arnica is used for bruises, sprains, broken bone swelling, muscle aches, wound healing, joint pain, and inflammation..
Arnica-based products provide natural pain relief and works as an anti-inflammatory.

Methylsulfonylmethane, or, MSM provides the body with essential sulfur. Sulfur helps the healing and repair processes of tissues. Joint pain caused by conditions like arthritis, sports, exercise, and repetitive use injuries, benefit from MSM.

Immune Boosters

Your Personal Defense System

Your immune system is your very own personal defense system. It works to protect you from viruses, funguses, bacteria and parasites, pollens, drugs, insect venoms and chemicals in food.

Age, stress, and poor nutrition can sap our immune system of its effectiveness. Daily exposure to environmental pollutants, stress, processed foods, and viruses all challenge our immune systems. An overload of antibiotics, antacids, or immunizations also affects our immune system balance.

Foods that stress or immune system include: sugar, white bread, white rice, alcohol, soda drinks, processed foods.

Nutritional deficiencies greatly hinder our immune system. A nutritional (whole food) diet is critical to your long term health. To increase our nutritional intake choose locally grown fruits and vegetables **preferably** organic.

Drink plenty of clean water (**not** tap water with fluoride and/or chlorine) and not plastic-bottled water. A good house filter is the "Pure" filter or a reverse osmosis filtration system.

Detox teas help support the immune system and you can find them at your local health food store.

Herbs like astragals, and dandelion also strengthen the immune system.

Detox

Hydrotherapy

Since the days of the ancient Egyptians and Romans, one tried and true method of boosting immunity and easing aches and pains has been hydrotherapy. Hydrotherapy uses water to treat pains, injuries, and illnesses.

A great way to treat minor aches and pains, as well as promote circulation and energy, is hydrotherapy. Hydrotherapy uses both hot and cold water to treat aches and pains as well as immune system boosting. Hot water increases blood flow to the skin surface.

Cold water directs the blood inward toward the internal organs and the core of the body. Alternating hot and cold water increases blood flow and speeds up circulation. It brings fresh oxygenated blood and nutrients to the organs and glands and carries away toxins. To increase circulation and detox internal organs just. Start with water, as hot as you can **comfortably** stand. Then, finish with cold water, as cold as you can stand.

Hydro therapy is used to treat cancer, kidney problems, aches and pains, and tumors. It is helpful to use clean, filtered water. You can get an inexpensive shower filter that lasts up to six months from home depot.

Popular energy drinks and caffeine-infused pills that claim to boost energy are full of harmful chemicals. These products may help in the short-term, but soon after, you'll feel sluggish... Instead of putting these toxins into your body why not try the holistic approach.

Detoxifying Foot Pads

There *are* natural ways to detox! There is sauna (sweating is a terrific detox) or sea salt/baking soda baths then bundle up to sweat out the toxins, juicing, herbal teas and my least favorite, but sometimes appropriate, is fasting.

Or you can Detox while you sleep!
Sounds easy enough, right? That's
because it is. Detox pads are a great way
to detoxify your body! The detox foot
pads that you place on the bottom of
your feet before you go to sleep really
do work and you get a great night's
sleep too!

These adhesive footpads are the
culmination of centuries of knowledge,
known to the Japanese, and passed
down through generations. Ingredients
such as distilled bamboo vinegar pulls
toxins from the bod. Naturally cleansing
your organs through the nerve endings
in your foot.

Be sure to use foot pads that are all natural and contain no harsh chemicals or animal ingredients.

Check "My Favorite Things" section for more information on a trusted brand!

The importance of cleansing our internal bodies of chemicals, toxins, and heavy metals cannot be overstated. So many people just don't know how these toxins affect their everyday life and their future health! So eliminate these stored toxins from your body through regular cleansing.

What I try to teach people is how easy it is to heal the body by activating your own self-healing mechanism. In years of practice and research, I've seen and experienced the benefits of keeping the body detoxified. This is the real "**secret**" to good health. This, along with a nutritional diet, is the easiest and fastest method of improving health and staying healthy.

We accumulate toxins in our daily life so the need to detox on a regular basis is profound. Sometimes the task is overwhelming but you can keep things simple by using these natural detoxing methods that will greatly improve how you look and feel. Oh, and don't forget the health benefits!

Food

Fermented Soy

There is a lot of conflicting information on soy. But, there are too many benefits to overlook this tasty, healthy food! Soy is one of my favorite foods for hormone balancing! This makes soy a great choice for pre-menopausal women. Here are some great reasons to include soy in your diet.. Some examples of health-promoting fermented soy foods include: Natto, miso, tempeh, and my favorite fermented soy — sake! Organic is the best choice.

Natto is actually a phenomenal food. Natto is very high in vitamin K2. Vitamin K2 and vitamin D together provide a large number of significant health benefits, such as improving bone density, reducing your risk of heart disease and cancer, and helping ease menopause symptoms. You can usually find Natto in your local health food store or an Asian market.

Miso supplies the digestive tract with beneficial bacteria know as probiotics. Probiotics help digestion, strengthen the immune system, helping to fight infection, synthesize, and assimilate nutrients necessary for good health and anti-aging.

The protein and fiber in **Tempeh** help to keep blood sugar levels under control. One serving of tempeh contains more fiber than most peoples consume in whole day and is an excellent source of health-promoting probiotics. Fiber is essential for a healthy digestive tract as well as preventing many chronic diseases.

Heart Healthy Foods

Your heart is like the battery of a car. You need to keep it charged to get you everywhere you need to go. Making some smart food choices is a simply way to make sure your heart is operating at optimum level

Smart Choices to Protect Your Heart
A diet low in saturated and trans fats, salt, processed and refined foods can help keep blood pressure down and drastically cut your risk for heart disease.

Fruits and vegetables, high-fiber foods, whole-grains, fish, and skinless turkey or chicken are excellent options. Garlic contain more than 30 different anti-carcinogens.

Garlic lowers serum cholesterol, blood pressure, triglycerides, blood fats, and helps dissolve blood clots (preventing heart attacks and strokes, and may even reverse arterial blockage caused by atherosclerosis.

The following foods are all good for your heart. Remember, always choose organic whenever possible:

Cold water fish: salmon, trout, tuna, and anchovies

Skinless poultry: turkey and chicken

Raw nuts and seeds

High fiber cereals

Whole grains: barley, brown rice, and

steel-cut oats

Onions and garlic

Edamame and tofu

Ginger

Olive oil

Avocado

Green and black tea

Even dark chocolate is good for your
heart!
The flavanoids in chocolate relax blood
vessels circulation and reduce platelet
activation. Plus, you can enjoy knowing
that dark chocolate has antioxidants.

Organic vs Natural

Let's clear up the Confusion between Organic, Natural or Conventional.
Two of the most popular buzzwords are: organic and natural. What's the difference? It is time to clear up the confusion of organic, natural and conventional.

Natural

"Natural" indicates a lack of **added** chemical pesticides, herbicides, or other synthetic additives to the crops but you **will** still find these chemicals in the product, because they are absorbed into the plants from the soil. Just to be clear, Natural soil is **not free** of chemicals or harmful fertilizers. Herbicides, insecticides, and synthetic fertilizers are carcinogenic that are absorbed by crops and into our bodies when eaten.

Certified Organic

In organic farming no genetically modified seeds, pesticides or other chemicals are used. Before a producer may qualify to be "Certified Organic", the land on which he grows or raises livestock must be free from chemicals for a period of two years prior to certification.

Organic crops are safe because they are grown without chemical fertilizers, pesticides, herbicides, or other chemicals so they do not absorb these toxic chemicals from the soil.

Organic farmers make use of crop-rotation and other traditional methods to keep the soil fertile and the crops free of pests.

Organic foods are not irradiated (treated with radiation to increase shelf life) a common practice in the conventional food industry today.

Organic products have more minerals, protein and flavorful than non-organic. Organic poultry and beef get chemical free feed

Convention (chemical) farming

Chemical farming has hidden costs that include: subsidies to corporate farmers, environmental damage, and health hazards. Managing soil quality is the foundation of organic farming. It is good for the environment, the earth, and our health. Chemical farming with pesticides, herbicides, and other chemicals contaminates the groundwater. Chemical farming pollutes the air and mono-cropping leaves the soil lacking in natural minerals and nutrients. This requires more chemicals to grow crops and higher concentrations of these chemicals get into the crops from the soil and from above ground crop dusting. Then consumed by us to add to toxic accumulation in the body. The risk of antibiotic resistance, and the risk of new viruses and bacteria damage to vital organs and the immune system, are all problems related to chemical farming Genetically engineered (GMO) products are a threat to human health because of the increased cancer risks but this is a common practice in conventional farming. Another major risk from genetically-manipulated foods (GMO) is the possibility that regular exposure to foreign DNA and RNA material inserted into these foods could cause allergic reactions or autoimmune diseases.

Irradiation (radioactive treatment) is another common practice in conventional farming and it is harmful because it changes the structure of the food's DNA and depletes the nutritional value. Microwaves use radioactive waves that change the DNA of food and deplete nutritional value as well. This is a good reason not to use them or at least use them less!

When you buy non-organic foods or processed and packaged foods, you are buying chemically-treated, possibly irradiated, and genetically modified food. In other words: nutritionally-void, empty-calorie food. That leaves you always hungry because your body is craving nutrients.

Buying local organic foods (and honey) will help relieve allergies and avoids trucking which creates better prices and helps the environment! Less trucks on the road is good for everyone (except maybe the truckers). A good source for all of these products is at your local farmers market and you can find great deals at closing time!

Here is where I feel it is important to point out the significant link, between all the pollutants and toxins we are subjected to and absorb, **with** the ramped outbreak of cancer and autoimmune diseases. I believe is the cause. I have had older people say to me we never worried about organic and my reply to them is that everything was organic when you grew up. These toxic chemicals, pesticides, plastics and pollutants were not around when you grew up. People grew their own food or hunted and fished (the waters were not so polluted then) so proportions of disease was not so epic

Cleaning Fruits and Veggies the Safe Way!

Fruits and vegetables need to be cleaned before being consumed. **Even organic**. I suggest diluted grapefruit seed extract, or, GSE. GSE will safely wash away the residue from environmental toxins. As always, I recommend organic.

When taken internally GSE has the extraordinary ability to perform against a wide variety of viruses, bacteria, funguses and parasites. GSE stimulates the immune system and is gentle, yet preserves the integrity of your intestinal bacteria. GSE helps **alkalize the body**. Disease cannot live in an alkaline environment. Cancer dies in a pH of 8.0.

When you eat food that is acid-forming such as meat, sugar, and white flour these foods create an acid environment within the body. GSE is very effective at low concentrations; a little goes a long way.

GSE is also a great surface cleaner and water purifier

Fruits and Vegetables – Natures Defense Enhancers.

Fruits are a major weapon against disease and have their best healing and nutritional effects when eaten alone.

Fruit and vegetables can accelerate body detoxification. For best energy conversion and cleaning benefits, eat fruit before noon. A great and easy way to enjoy a daily dose of fruit is a fruit smoothie with honey — one of my favorites!

Cooked fruit changes its' properties from alkalizing to acid forming in the body. Eat organic whenever possible. Pesticides and chemicals are absorbed

by the plants and enter the body
rapidly.
The healing power of vegetables works
both raw and cooked.

Natural Sweeteners

Natural sugars like those found in fruits and vegetables are necessary for a healthy immune system because they support beneficial micro flora in the gut.

Natural Sweeteners

Organic honey is composed of trace enzymes, minerals, vitamins, and amino acids and contains flavanoids and antioxidants that eliminate free radicals. The darker the honey, the better. Organically harvested honey is always better because there are no hormones, pesticides, or synthetic preservatives added.

Organic molasses contains a variety of minerals and is an excellent source of iron, calcium, cooper, manganese, potassium and magnesium.

Natural organic syrup contains much fewer calories, has higher concentrations of key minerals for health and is an excellent source of manganese and zinc. These sweeteners are high anti-oxidants to help you body process the sugars and are chuck full of digestive enzymes.

Artificial

Sweeteners

Artificial Sweeteners

Aspartame is the most common sweetener used in diet soda and low-cal or low-sugar products. Studies have found that drinking diet soda may increase your risk of developing diabetes.

Aspartame becomes toxic to brain cells when mixed with food color. It enters the brain and creates neurotoxins at the brain center. Food color is a common ingredient in packaged, processed foods and drinks.

Sucralose, also known as **Splenda**,. Splenda may not penetrate the blood brain barrier as aspartame does, but Splenda can adversely affect the body in many ways because it is a *chemical substance* and not a *natural* sugar. Sucralose is processed from sugar using chlorine. Sucralose contains small amounts of potentially dangerous substances such as: heavy metals, arsenic, and methanol.

Although agave has become the popular natural sweetener alternative, it is not our best choice because Agave is close to 90% fructose.

Protein

Protein

Your body must have protein to heal. Protein is essential to our bodies' normal functions. Protein helps in producing enzymes and hormones, maintaining fluid balance, and regulating such vital functions as building antibodies against infection, and blood clotting. Protein is a source of energy, the major source of building material for muscles, blood, skin, hair, nails and internal organs (the heart and brain).

But, Americans consume too much protein. Too much protein irritates the immune system. Too much protein causes fluid imbalance which results in the loss of calcium and other minerals through the urine.

Animal protein contributes to osteoporosis, heart disease, and increased cholesterol deposits while **vegetable protein lowers cholesterol deposits.**

When your consume more protein than the recommended level, as you might do if following a high protein diet, it puts additional stress on the kidney.The kidney's main purpose is to take away excess protein that your body is not utilizing. By eating excess protein, your kidney will need to work overtime, causing strain and dehydration. Protein metabolism requires extra water for utilization and elimination of its by-products.

Exercising individuals are at an increased risk for dehydration, the additional strain of protein waste excretion may further promote dehydration, kidney problems, nausea, and headaches. High blood pressure is a side effect that can come about over time due to a diet high in protein.

Excess protein leads to an increase in the loss of calcium through the urinary tract. Chronic calcium loss, due to excess protein intake, is of particular concern to women over 35 because it may increase the risk of osteoporosis.

A high protein diet may result in weight loss but this is mostly water weight, brought about by dehydration.

Daily Protein Requirements

Daily protein needs vary for each individual. The contributing factors to protein needs include age, weight, and lifestyle. Generally speaking a healthy adult needs around 0.36 grams per pound of body weight.

Example: a 100 pound healthy adult would want to consume 36 grams of protein a day.

Carbs

Carbohydrates = Brain Fuel

Flip through a magazine and you will find the latest and greatest low- or no-carb diets craze! These diets do not actually work long term. A reduced carbohydrate diet will help you lose weight but, it is purely water weigh, and they slow your metabolism? When your metabolism slows you stop losing weight.

Carbohydrates, the right kind, are essential to human life.

Not all Carbs are Created Equal

Carbohydrates provide energy and regulate glucose in the bloodstream. Glucose is the blood-sugar obtained from starches and sugar and usually is the only fuel used by brain cells. You read that right—your brain needs carbohydrates!

Neurons in the brain cannot store glucose, so they depend on the bloodstream to deliver a constant supply. By dramatically reducing or completely slashing your carbohydrate intake, you are robbing your brain of essential nutrients. With diets like South Beach, Zone, and Atkins you will probably experience headaches, fatigue, increased forgetfulness, or inability to focus.

Healthy carbohydrates are those carbohydrates that digest slowly to provide your brain with the fuel it needs for energy, normal body function, and to keep you focused. Healthy carbohydrates an important part of a healthy diet.

The healthiest source of carbohydrates include unprocessed whole grains, vegetables, fruits and beans.

Unhealthier sources of carbohydrates include white bread, sodas, and processed or refined foods. These carbohydrates may contribute to weigh gain, interfere with weight loss, and promote diabetes and heart disease.

Great Grains

Great Grains!

Give sprouted grain bread a try. The benefits include, low glycemic index, low saturated fat, high fiber, high protein source, helps the body cleanse itself, enhances the availability of vitamins A, B, and C, iron, potassium and calcium. Protein and vitamin contents can increase 300 to 600 percent

For the gluten sensitive you can use the no gluten, or low gluten sprouted wheat bread option. Sprouts' enzymes effectively break down gluten and difficult-to-digest wheat components. Trade Joes carries an organic sprouted grain bread that is very tasty!

Sprouted wheat bread has a low

glycemic index and does not cause post-meal blood-sugar levels or blood-fat counts to spike so this makes sprouted bread a good choice for a diabetic.

Whole grains also provide your body much-needed fiber, a nutrient missing from many of our diets.

Mental Health

Quiet Time

Finding a quiet moment for yourself everyday can be a very healing activity. I know everyone's lives are full and busy, but if you do not take time for *you*, then you can not be at your best.

A daily ritual of finding five minutes or more just for you can be helpful in many ways. You will sleep better, be in a better mood, be more tolerant, the world will look better and you will feel better!

Quiet time gives the body and mind time to relax and center. This is especially helpful when stress has taken hold causing agitation and the inability to get anything accomplished effectively.

Life can sometimes get so loud it drowns out your own better judgment. Taking a moment for some deep breathing can change your attitude and perspective.

By quieting your mind and focusing on your breath, stress lessens, endorphins are released, attention and memory improves, and pain eases.

Quiet time is your time! Take it! Your health, body, and mind deserve it!

Sleep Aids

Having Trouble Sleeping?

Sleep is very important to your health. It is the time when your boy rejuvenates, rebuilds, and replenishes.

Many people have trouble sleeping due to stress or anxiety. Thankfully, there is an all natural, non-sedative, non-habit forming remedy to ease you into a restful sleep.

Hyland's Calms Forte

Calms Forte relieves stress and relaxes your body with chamomile. It soothes nerves and edginess, easing you into a peaceful sleep. Unlike many prescription-sleep aids, you will wake alert and refreshed! Since it contains no sedatives, there's no risk for any foggy, groggy "hangover-feeling" in the morning. Calms Forte is non habit-forming. It is a homeopathic formula of all- natural ingredients that works without risk of dependency.

.

Hyland's Calms Tablets

Calms tablets provide relief to symptoms related to stress, nervousness, or nervous exhaustion. Calms Tablets have a soothing and calming effect to quiet irritated nerves and sooth away edginess. My personal favorite!

A fatigued person is accident-prone,

judgment impaired, irritable, moody, and more likely to make mistakes and bad decisions. Although the optimal hours of sleep each night vary by individual, most adults need seven to eight hours of sleep per night. Deep, restful, non-interrupted sleep is very important to staying healthy and fighting off disease.

Magnet Therapy

Another way to promote sleep is magnet therapy. Magnets can help improve sleep and circulation. Magnets help with pain management, the effects of aging, and for diabetics afflicted with tingling feet and hands.

Magnets work by stimulating and balancing the electromagnetic energy fields in the body, improving circulation, and promoting faster healing and general good health. According to Wolfgang Ludwig, Sc.D., Ph.D., Director of the Institute for Biophysics in Horb, Germany, "Magnetic field therapy has been used effectively in the treatment of:

Cancer

Rheumatoid disease

Infections and inflammations

Headaches and migraines

Insomnia and sleep disorders

Circulatory problems

Fractures and pain

Environmental stress."

Magnetic therapy devices range from small, simple magnets to large machines. Magnetic blankets and beds are available for the purposes of promoting sleep and reducing stress. I prefer the mattress pad magnets and magnetic jewelry.

Laughter, Music, Color Therapy

Laughter Therapy

Do you know that laughter actually exercises the liver?

There is a theory that people have laughed themselves healthy and even case studies documenting people healing from laughter!

Laughter causes the widening of the inner lining of blood vessels and increases blood flow.

Laughter lifts more than your spirits; it also boosts your immune response. Laughter lowers cortisol, an immune suppressor leading to a stronger immune system. Laughter seems to be an underlying factor in good health. A good reason to LOL.

Laughter promotes oxygen flow to the body. The physiological and psychological benefits are worth a little silliness! So be kind to your liver, immune system, and boost your mood! Maybe we should all try to surround ourselves with more beauty and laughter and reap the benefits. The quote "Laughter is the best medicine," is great advice to live by.

"Always laugh when you can. It is cheap medicine." Lord Byron

Music Therapy

Music therapy is a serious field of study. More than seventy colleges and universities have degree programs. Music is used to restore, maintain, and improve physical, physiological, and spiritual health and wellbeing.

Brain function physically changes in response to music. Heart rate and blood pressure are also responsive to the types of music that we listened to. Music can sharpen mental acuity, assist in relaxation or provide some relief from pain, through release of endorphins.

Ancient Greek philosophers believed that music could heal both the body and the soul. Native Americans used singing and chanting as part of their healing rituals. A 1993 study showed that college students improved their IQs by listening to Mozart's sonata.

Many cancer centers and hospitals use music therapy as part of a cancer-management program. Some music therapy services are covered by health insurance.

Music therapy is an automatic process of deep inner-healing set in motion through the right combinations of sounds.. Music sound therapy is an arrangement of sounds, in a specific order and design, to invoke different feelings that influence our DNA.

Music Therapy influences the immune system, blood pressure, pain perception, and heart and respiratory rates.

Music Therapy is used in labor and delivery, oncology, pain management, physical rehabilitation and pediatrics. When a blocked organ stops vibrating at a healthy frequency that results in some kind of illness. Music and light (color) therapy can break up, dissolve and release these blockages.

What you listen to matters. The next time you're down and you need a lift, listen to, or play some happy music. It can make an ordinary day extraordinary.

There is power in the spoken word (example: subliminal messaging and hypnosis). This is why lyrics are so important! You should know the words to the music you listen too!

Color Therapy

The use of Color is a holistic therapy that dates back thousands of years. Chromotherapy (color therapy) is a method of treatment that uses color to cure disease. It is a centuries old concept used successfully to cure various diseases. Color therapy has been used to kill bacteria and for healing T-cell leukemia for years. The effects of color therapy are non-invasive and can occur at a deep cellular level.

Color therapy aims to balance and enhance our body's energy by using the colors of the rainbow to help stimulate our body's own healing process.

Color therapy is a non-invasive therapy for adults, babies, children and animals.

Color affects energy, mood and can transform our lives.

.

Infrared sauna manufacturers are including color therapy in portable home saunas. The color therapy lights maximize the healing benefits of that sauna.

Turn your bath into a sensory experience that can stimulate, or relax, soothe, regenerate, and refresh with the color and scent of bath salts.

Indigo acts as a calming sedative. **Violet** sooths the internal organs, relaxing muscles and calming the nervous system.

Blue has a detoxifying effect to treat liver disorders and jaundice.

Green Is effective in ulcer treatment and bacterial infections because of its antiseptic properties.

Yellow has decongestant and antibacterial properties and invigorates both the digestive and lymphatic system.

Orange has anti-bacterial properties and provides relief for digestive discomforts.

Red improves circulation and stimulates red blood cell production

Color therapy can be incorporated into you daily life with the color of the cloths you wear, the color of the food you eat, color therapy bath salts, the colors you decorate your home with, the colors in nature, colored glassed that are filled with water and left in the sun for sun infused water you drink, or buy light therapy lamps and even the jewelry we wear. So have fun experimenting with color in your life!

Yoga

Yoga

You've probably heard that yoga is good for you. But, more importantly there are the specific health benefits you can expect to enjoy from doing yoga regularly.

Blood pressure. A consistent yoga practice decreases blood pressure through better circulation and oxygenation of the body.

Circulation. Yoga improves blood circulation to transport nutrients and oxygen throughout your body for healthier organs, skin, and brain.

Respiratory. Yoga decreases the respiratory rate through controlled breathing exercises.

Cardiovascular. Lower heart rate and improved oxygenation (both benefits of yoga) results in higher cardiovascular endurance.

Pain. Yoga lessens or eliminates pain, such as back pain with regular practice.

Aging. Yoga stimulates the detoxification process which delays the aging process.

Posture. With consistent practice, your posture will improve.

Energy. You will feel energized after your yoga session rather than tired.

Weight. Yoga improves metabolism to keep your weight in check and helps to reduce cellulite.

Sleep. Many find that they sleep much better with regular yoga practice.

Mood. Overall well-being, and mood improves with regular yoga practice.

Anxiety and Stress. The controlled breathing used in yoga helps to reduce anxiety.

Yoga calms the mind and energizes the body Yoga suits all levels of fitness, increases strength and flexibility. Yoga increases endorphins, promoting peace of mind and relaxation.

Kundalini Yoga is **not** about mastering and holding difficult exercises.
Basically, if you can breathe you can do Kundalini Yoga.
Kundalini yoga poses and postures stimulate glands, organs and quiet the mind. A couple of my favorite yoga CD's are: Kundalini Yoda with Grace and Strength featuring Carol Carlson and Kundalini Yoga with Gurnukh.

Home Care

Cookware

The foods you eat are important to overall health. But did you know that what you use to prepare your food can also contribute to your health, positively or negatively?

Aluminum Cookware

Large amounts of aluminum in the body can over time contribute to mental deterioration.

Studies now link Alzheimer's to aluminum.

The aluminum to which we are exposed comes from many sources. Dust, water, processed foods, cosmetics, many medicines, and food additives contain aluminum. Also, some brands of baking powders, baking soda, cake mixes, canned items, kitchenware, utensils, antacids, aluminum foil, and some drinking water can contain dangerous amounts of aluminum. Read labels before purchasing.

One of the kidney's jobs is to eliminate things like aluminum, but we overwork our kidneys with the wrong choices. Toxic amounts of aluminum can impair kidney function making healthy kidneys unhealthy over time. Aluminum not only has no recognized function in the body, but is also toxic.

Better Choices

It is best to eliminate aluminum consumption where and when ever possible. That includes aluminum foil and aluminum cans and aluminum cookware! Aluminum is a fairly soft metal that leaks aluminum into food.

Teflon pans release at **least six toxic** gases including **two carcinogens, two global pollutants, and MFA, a chemical lethal to humans at low doses**. When Teflon is heated these chemicals get drawn out of the pan and into your food. These chemicals lead to various hormonal disruptions. When your hormonal messages get disrupted then your testosterone (yes, women have testosterone that needs to be balanced too) and cortisol balances will be disrupted.

Since these chemicals are fat soluble, your body will place them into fat cells that are resistant to detoxing procedures. So when we are trying to lose stomach fat these fat soluble cells resist being broken down and to be eliminated. So we can't lose the fat because of all of these harmful chemicals

Think about this for a second. You're cooking food in Teflon pans that infuses your food with these harmful chemicals. There are much better choices! I will list some of those choices below.

Healthy Cookware Choices

Your choice of cookware — including cooking utensils — is important! Here are some healthier choices: Cast iron, stainless steel, Pyrex, Dutch ovens, crock pot, and pressure cookers.

Cooking in cast iron increases the dietary source of iron. Cast-iron cookware allows iron to leak onto your food as it cooks, beneficial especially to those suffering from anemia.

No Plastic Please

Bisphenol (BPA) is arguably one of the most disturbing hormonal disrupters that seeps into foods and liquids when stored in plastic. BPA stimulates the growth of cancer cells, is linked to behavioral changes, and altered immune function in young children.

Extreme temperatures (hot or cold), acidic conditions: soft drinks, coffee, citrus of any kind, vinegar-containing foods, tomatoes, pickles, or fatty foods and drinks (milk, salad dressing, meats, oils, peanut butters, shortening) absorb higher levels of BPA.

Plastic used for cooking or storing increases risks! Heating (in a hot car, microwave, left out in the sun) or freezing greatly increases risks.

Plastic can be found in our clothing, toys, utensils, dishes, food containers, baby bottles, or "Sippy" cups, pacifiers, teething toys, and the list goes on.

Some alternative suggestions for storing: Pyrex, corning ware, and glass containers. You can find some great air tight glass storing dishes at Costco.

Also use stainless steel utensils whenever possible rather than plastic.

Paper Products

Paper towels, paper cups and plates, waxed paper, facial tissues, napkins, sanitary napkins and toilet paper contain formaldehyde and dioxin. If you are going to use paper towels, it's better to use **unbleached** brown paper towels toilet paper. A better choice is cloth napkins whenever possible.

Glass or stainless steel are better choices for drink ware. Do not use aluminum or plastic. I buy water in glass bottles (like Voss) to reuse and refill. But, so, many online retailers and Costco sell ceramic, glass and stainless steel containers for people on the move.

I am happy to say that I have seen organic kids' toys, bottles, cloths etc. in a lot of retail stores recently so we are making headway on finding healthier choices in more places now. Yeah!

Because I believe this can't be over-stated I repeat, it is important to point out the significant link between all the pollutants and toxins we are subjected to and absorb to the ramped numbers of cancer and autoimmune today.

Clothing

Cotton Verses Synthetic Clothing

Fabric may not be the first thing that comes to mind when you think about living a healthier lifestyle, but it definitely should be. Most people don't realize that synthetic fabrics are teeming with chemicals and dyes making them a potential health hazard because they are absorbed through the skin or inhaled directly

Most synthetic fabrics are treated with chemicals. That includes towels and bed linens, and most clothing. These chemicals leach into the environment, leaving an impact on groundwater, wildlife, air and soil.

.

"The use of man-made chemicals is increasing, and at the same time we have warning signals that a variety of wildlife and human health problems are becoming more prevalent," says Dr. Richard Dixon, Head of the World Wildlife Federation (WWF) Scotland. "It is reckless to suggest there is no link between the two and give chemicals the benefit of the doubt. Urgent action is needed to replace hazardous chemicals with safer alternatives especially in clothing and other consumer products."

Organic, all-natural fabrics like cotton, wool and linen may be the safest options when it comes to your health

Chemical in Your Clothing?

Perafluorinated chemicals (PFCs) are added to clothing because it makes them wrinkle-free and last longer.

Formaldehyde is a product used on fabric to prevent shrinkage. Long-term exposure to low levels of formaldehyde may cause respiratory difficulty, eczema, nasal and lung cancer.

Petrochemical dyes used for color pollute waterways.

.

Nylon and polyester is made from petrochemicals. Petrochemicals are chemicals made from petroleum (crude oil) and natural gas and they are linked to kidney and liver damage with repeated (dermal) skin and oral exposure because these build up in the fatty tissue of the liver, brain, kidneys and spleen.

Rayon is made from wood pulp that is treated with sulfuric acid (sulfuric acid is a strong chemical that is corrosive and can cause buns and tissue damage when it comes in contact with the skin, and caustic soda (highly corrosive that can be irritating to the skin, eyes, and gastrointestinal tract..

Dyes in fabrics often come from heavy metals and accumulate in the body. The chemicals used in synthetic clothing is linked to health problems including:

cancer, immune system damage, behavioral problems and hormone disruption.

Without knowing it, parents are exposing their children to toxic chemicals in clothing that could have serious future consequences for their health and the environment.
Children are usually more vulnerable to the effects of chemicals than adults.
Be especially careful with babies bedding, clothing, and car seats.
Now you can rate your choices online before you purchase.

Synthetic Fibers to Avoid

If at all possible, it's best to stay away from **anything labeled: static-resistant, wrinkle-resistant, permanent-press, no-iron, stain-proof or moth-repellant and** the following fabrics: **acrylic, polyester, rayon, acetate, triacetate, and nylon** in lieu of more natural options. Natural fabrics like cotton, linen, wool, cashmere, silk, and hemp. Natural fabrics allow the skin to breathe.

Organic clothing is made from organic cotton that has been cultivated according to the guidelines of organic farming.
Organic fabrics are becoming more widely available and can be found in

health food markets, specialty shops, some department stores, and online.

Wash and dry all new garments s before wearing.

Do not use conventional dryer sheets, as they are loaded with toxic chemicals.

Wash your clothing in non-toxic detergent and seek out environmentally friendly dry-cleaners that do not use harsh, toxic chemicals.

Buy American whenever possible, lets' keep Americans working please!

Footwear

Thanks to organic and eco-friendly companies, we're getting closer to being able to dress organically and naturally from head to toe. Go barefoot whenever possible it is great for the sole too.
Even some footwear is made with organic materials
Toms' is my favorite eco-friendly shoemaker! It's also a great source of giving back – for every pair sold, a free pair is given to a child in need!

Most athletic shoes use rubber which is not biodegradable, which means it will sit in a landfill for eternity. Although organic shoes are harder to find, and you do not have as many choices, it is worth the effort because remember the skin absorbs toxins and the feet have hundreds of nerve endings that absorb these toxins.

Commercially used leather is subjected to tanning, keeping the material from biodegrading. The tanning process involves mineral salts, formaldehyde, coal tar derivatives, and dyes, some of which are cyanide-based. Most of the leather in the United States is chrome-tanned so search for untreated (organic) leather when you can.

Purchasing footwear made of organic cotton, linen, and canvas is a healthier choice for you and the earth.

Ban the Stinky Feet

Wear natural fiber shoes to avoid stinky foot odor. Go barefoot whenever possible and let those toes breath.

Clean Air in the Home

According to the American Medical Association (AMA), 50% of all illnesses may be caused or aggravated by poor indoor air quality. Houseplants are our often-overlooked helpers in ridding the air of pollutants and toxins. Houseplants are our most effective tool in keeping household air clean and pure.

Improve indoor air quality with these plants. These plants are effective at increasing oxygen and clearing out toxins for cleaner breathing air. Research has shown that these plants are the most effective as an all-around protector in counteracting off-gassed chemicals from furniture and house paint etc.

Aloe Plant helps to monitor the air quality in your home. The plant can help clear the air of pollutants and harmful chemicals such as those in chemical cleaning products.

English Ivy is the best air-filtering house plan because it is the most effective plant when it comes to absorbing formaldehyde (furniture out-gasses formaldehyde).

Rubber Tree is a low- maintenance powerful toxin eliminator and air purifier.

Peace Lily help reduce toxins in the air.

Sansevieria (Snake Plant) absorbs carbon dioxide and releases oxygen during the night (while most plants do during the day).

Bamboo Palm is particularly effective at cleaning out benzene. Benzene is a component of products derived from coal and petroleum. Benzene is used in the manufacturing of plastics.

Philodendrum another great plant for absorbing formaldehyde.

Spider Plant is effective at fighting pollutants like benzene, formaldehyde, and carbon monoxide.

Also, a good hepa-filter air cleaner can help to keep indoor air safe. Negative ions in your air filter not only help keep the air clean but lifts your mood. Science has proven that particles floating in the air are doing so because they are positively charged. This includes dust, pollen, toxic residues and emissions coming from household furnishings, rugs, construction materials, viruses, bacteria and germs. These all present a potential health problem because they are floating in our air and being inhaled. These toxins become positively charged by static electricity, from walking across carpets or from recycled air and heating systems. Negative ions help reduce floating particles.

Clean air helps us reach a more toxic-free body.

Additional tips to consider for helping to keep your home clean and toxin free:

- Change air conditioning filters every two to three months.

- Use exhaust fans in kitchens and bathrooms to vent air outdoors.

- Have ducts for forced-air furnaces cleaned.

- Don't keep your recycling items (newspapers, rags, cans or bottles) inside your home. They can release toxic vapors.

- Use non- toxic household cleaners.. Do not mix cleaning products. Use natural cleaners, such as vinegar, lemon juice, or baking soda.

- Paint can release trace gases for months after you apply it. Try to use paint without volatile organic compounds (VOCs).
- Many furnishings contain formaldehyde. When shopping for new furniture or cabinets, try to buy those that are made of solid hardwood. Avoid particleboard-based products, which usually have a wood-veneer finish that contains formaldehyde.
- Make sure wood stoves and fireplaces have tight-fitting doors. Check flues and chimneys for cracks that could allow fumes into your house.
- Check houseplants for mold.

- Bathe and groom pets often to reduce dander.

Easing Allergy Symptoms

Quercetin

Quercetin bioflavonoid is a natural antioxidant found in citrus fruits, onions, apples, parsley, tea, tomatoes, broccoli, and lettuce. Allergy sufferers, can use quercetin supplements, about 1,000 milligrams a day. Those with liver disease shouldn't use quercetin.

People who eat foods rich in omega-3 fatty acids are less likely to suffer allergy symptoms. Horseradish, chili peppers or hot mustard act as natural decongestants.

Stinging Nettle

 Stinging Nettle inhibits the body's ability to produce histamine. Studies have shown that taking about 300 milligrams daily will offer relief for most people.

Eating locally grown foods and honey work to reduce allergy symptoms. Your local farmer's market is a great place to buy these — it saves the environment from trucking products to market.

Going Green

Tips for Reducing Your Electric Bill

We're all looking to save money; where better to start than in your own home? Electricity costs are rising dramatically, but there are ways to save money while also lessening our carbon footprint.

Where to Start

Think of the major electricity drainers in your home. Some appliances may pop into your mind: refrigerator, freezer, washer, dryer, and dishwasher. By taking small steps everyday, you can reduce the amount of energy utilized by every one of these appliances.

If you keep your refrigerator and freezer full it takes less energy to operate. This helps to keep everything cold. For example, I keep glass bottles of water in the refrigerator and bags of ice in the freezer when it's getting low on food.

Peak times for energy usage are in the midmorning hours: 8:00 a.m. – 10:00 a.m. and afternoon/evening hours: 4:30 p.m. – 8:00 p.m. This makes sense, these hours are when most people are waking up, getting ready for work and coming home form work, cooking dinner, and taking showers.

How do you avoid the Peak Hour Trap? Plan ahead. If you use the washer and dryer in the early morning hours you can avoid the peak hour trap. Line dry your cloths whenever possible. The same rule applies to the dishwasher. By using the dishwasher at non-peak times, you can cut energy costs.

The other great tip I got years ago is to unplug everything that is not in use. You will be amazed how much lower you bill will be! Unplug unused appliances like blenders, coffee makers, TVs, etc.

Try a smart power strip! These smart strips have several outlets to plug in various devices. When the items are not in use, just flip the switch. Some retailers sell power strips that have an automatic shut off timer. Set the timer for when you're not at home, and watch your usage and energy bill drop. I guarantee you will see a major difference if you just try these money saving tips for a couple months.

Another useful tip? Why make use of natural light instead of artificial? Open your shades and blinds — let the sun in! In the winter, keep shades that are on the shady side of the house closed and shades that are facing the sun, open. Then, do the opposite in the summer. These may sound a little too time consuming, but I promise you will be surprised how big a difference they make! You'll be amazed at the extra money you'll have and not to mention you'll be helping the environment!

Household Cleansers

My recommendation for greener cleaning is a vinegar and baking soda combination. White vinegar is great for cleaning, even laundry. Vinegar is a with vinegar. It will fizz, showing it is working. My favorite way to clean away the bacteria and germs and deodorize naturally.natural cleanser and deodorizer and is effective for killing most mold, bacteria, and germs. It even works on windows! Just use the ratio of half water and half vinegar for a streak free clean! Baking soda's neutralizing action makes it an effective deodorizer. Added to the water when doing laundry, baking soda stabilizes the pH level, enhancing the detergent's effectiveness. Baking soda may also be added to swimming pool water to balance the pH and keep the water clear. For showers and bath tubs, sprinkle baking soda and then spray

Do you suffer from sensitive skin? Not to worry! Non-toxic liquid laundry soap will keep you from itching or getting a rash. Non-toxic soaps are also better for the environment. They are easy to find in Costco, Whole Foods, or most health food stores.

Another tip: use table salt in cold water for the first wash of new colored clothes to keep them from running and fading.

Helpful Tips

Had An X-Ray Lately?

We are exposed to radiation every day of our lives from natural sources (the sun, vegetation, even our tap water) and man-made sources (x-rays, microwaves, and the television). How do you clear your system and protect your body from these harmful rays? It is as easy as taking a bath!

Baking soda and sea salt baths help to clear lymphatic congestion and radiation from your body. Salt is high in alkaline, assisting in the cleansing of your body and removing of toxins. Plus, you'll be able to take time out and relax!

Baths are wonderfully healing, and it is

easy to make your own homemade, detox baths with only two ingredients:

- 1 lb box of baking soda (aluminum free if possible)
- 1 lb sea salt (Himalayan Mineral Salt)

Use warm to hot water, soak, and enjoy! Bundle up after your bath. The sweat will help rid your body of harmful toxins.

For Coffee Lovers

Is drinking coffee good for you? Recent evidence suggests that the good outweighs the bad.

Coffee is rich in antioxidants and recent medical research suggests that drinking coffee in moderation can reduced the risk of illnesses and improve mental performance.

Here are some of coffee's health benefits:

- Increases mental focus
- Reduces the risk of cirrhosis of the liver lover by 60-80%
- Protects your body against Parkinson's disease
- Reduces the risk of Alzheimer's
- Reduces the rates of age-related cognitive decline
- Great source for antioxidants
- Increases energy
- Increases metabolism

Enjoy your morning java in moderation without guilt! But remember organic whenever possible.

Help Prevent Breast Cancer

With pink ribbons, which are now synonymous with breast cancer awareness, everywhere these days it is shocking to learn that some cosmetics companies are not treating their customers with care. Estee Lauder has been trumpeting its commitment to breast cancer awareness through promotions and pink ribbon campaigns, while at the same time lobbying against legislation in California requiring cosmetics companies to notify the state when they use chemicals linked to cancer and birth defects.

Awareness about early detection and treatment options is important. But, when one in eight women will be diagnosed with breast cancer, we need to get chemicals linked to cancer out of products we use every day – including cosmetics from pink ribbon companies.

The President's Cancer Panel concluded in its May 2010 report that many **cancers are linked to environmental exposures**. Lax regulations around toxic chemicals allow the use of known carcinogens and hormone disruptors in common products like cosmetics, hair, and body care products. Higher estrogen exposures throughout a woman's life can increase her risk of breast cancer, according to the latest scientific evidence.

So please, be sure to check the products you use on a daily basis. We can be natural, organic, healthy, *and* beautiful!

It is important to note here that there are finally reports out that link **mammograms to increased risk of cancer due to radiation exposure**. Self-examination is encouraged along with proper diet and personal care products. This information has been around for years so I am glad to see these reports now getting media attention.

Medical Cabinet
Musts

Medicine cabinet musts to promote health and wellness.

Colloidal Silver

Colloidal silver supports the natural defense system of the body, and is a powerful natural antibiotic. Various studies show colloidal silver to be able to kill over 650 micro-organisms.
It is effective to ward off colds, flu, and infections when used orally.
Use topically by spraying onto cuts, burns, skin infections or acne. I use it to heal cuts fast and relieve pain, as well as clean a wound and keep it from getting infected. It is great for burns, lessens pain within minutes, and speeds up healing time and keeps THE AREA clean from infection. It is painless and

works fast! I am never without it for an all-around cure.

My family now relies on me to have it for anything that comes up where ever we are. I keep a bottle of colloidal silver in the medicine cabinet and a spray bottle of diluted colloidal silver in my purse.

Also, I spray it on my dogs if they get sick or have a wheezing spell (especially during allergy season) and it works great!

I recommend the high parts per minute (PPM

It has been reported to be effective in fighting against: AIDS, acne, allergies, arthritis, athletes' foot, boils, burns, cystitis, diabetes, eczema, hay fever, indigestion, parasitic infections, psoriasis, ringworm, warts and yeast infections.

Organic Feminine Hygiene Products
Tampons are usually made from rayon. The word Rayon means more dioxins. Dioxins are nasty, nasty compounds. Dioxins are produced through the chlorine bleaching of wood pulp. Dioxin, a toxic carcinogen, is a by-product of all chlorine bleaching methods. Dioxin collects in the fatty tissues which makes detoxing difficult. Published scientific reports have shown that even low levels of dioxins are linked to cancer, endometriosis, low

sperm counts and immune system suppression.

Organic, 100% cotton non-chlorine bleached tampons (dioxin free) do not contain synthetics or chemical additives or the pesticide residues used on traditional cotton.

The first tampons were made of all-cotton but in the 1970's, chemicals were added and toxic shock syndrome (TSS) increased. Switching to an organic, all-cotton, and lower-absorbency tampon will reduce the risk of TSS. Trader Joe's and Whole Foods carry organic tampons or you can order them online.

White Willow Bark

White willow bark comes from a tree indigenous to Europe and Asia

In the medical community, white willow bark has been used for centuries. White willow bark has been used as a traditional treatment to relieve pain and fevers in China since 500 B.C. Ancient Egyptians used white willow for inflammation of the joints

But in the 1800's Salicin was removed from white willow bark to make the first aspirin, then because this was expensive and time-consuming, a scientist in the 1850's created synthetic salicin. It was an acid, harder on the stomach. Some users developed stomach ulcers and bleeding. These are the kind of side effects man made medicines have but white willow bark can be used without the risk of damaging the stomach's lining — as aspirin can do for pain (headaches), fever and inflammation..

Cayenne Pepper

Cayenne pepper (known as red pepper) is said to have the ability to boost circulation and increase heart action and even stopped a heart attack.

Suggested usage if a heart attack occurs: Take a teaspoon of extract or a teaspoon of Cayenne pepper in a glass of hot water every fifteen minutes until help arrives or the crisis passes. Let's hope no one has to try this out but good information to have stored just in case.

Neti Pot

Neti Pots are great for flushing the sinuses, and keeping them clean and clear. Saltwater can rinse away pollen grains and help treat allergies and sinus congestion.

Pour a quarter teaspoon of non-iodized table salt or a couple drops of colloidal silver or even grapefruit seed extract and lukewarm water into the pot. Follow directions on the Neti Pot.

Use your pot twice a day during allergy season.

Castor Oil Packs

Castor Oil packs are a great way to relieve aches and pains and draw out toxins. Pour castor oil onto organic cotton or organic flannel and place over the site of the ailment or pain. Apply heat with a heating pad for an hour or two. Castor oil packs can be used to improve elimination and circulation of the lymphatic system. Castor oil packs have been used for thousands of years, but grew in popularity in the mid 1900's. Edgar Cayce, known as the "Sleeping Prophet", recommended them for healing medical conditions.

Menopause

Perimenopause is a time of fluctuating hormones leading to menopause. During which time the production of estrogen and progesterone begins to decline resulting in irregular period. Some women experience perimenopause as early as their late thirties and can last from two to five years.

A common **misconception** in conventional medicine is that this is a problem of low estrogen levels.

The first hormone that begins to decline is progesterone. This creates an imbalance between estrogen and progesterone. Since a woman is estrogen dominant as she enters perimenopause, improving progesterone and estrogen balance should be the focus. Diet can improve hormonal balance with foods like soy,broccoli, kale and flax. Avoid dairy, beef, caffeine, alcohol and refined sugar because these feed estrogen dominance and worsen symptoms.

Some symptoms of perimenopause include:
Heavier periods or changes to the cycle length.
Bleeding between periods
Mood swings
Foggy Thinking and Forgetfulness
Low Thyroid function (weight gain)
Hot flashes and night sweats
Headaches
Heart Palpatations
Breast Tenderness

There are natural, safe and effective ways to support the transition into menopause. They include diet, herbs, lifestyle choices, natural remedies, exercise, rest and relaxation.

Phytotherapy is the use of herbs to relieve symptoms. The benefit of using herbs for menopause symptoms is the way they adapt to our unique individual needs. With herb your body can access as little or as much as needed. Unlike prescription drugs that overwhelm the body's natural response.

Herbs that can relieve symptons include black cohosh, alfalfa, fennel, licorice root, don quai, and chaste berries. Experiment with these to see which ones help you. The most effective herbs and plants for menopause have been identified as black cohosh, kudzu, red clover, passionflower, chasteberry, wild yam, **soy**. Soy is one of the most widely used plant-based menopause remedies (as stated previously organic and fermented soy is what I recommend). Soy is the reason that Japanese women in Japan rarely experience menopause symptoms. Soy is a staple in the Japanese diet (Miso is a fermented soy as is Sake). Adding organic fermented soy to your diet not only alleviates the perimenopause symptoms but reduces the risk of breast cancer, heart disease, and osteoporosis.

Yoga can help ease your transition by stabilizing hormones, relieving stress, and balancing the endocrine system. The regular practice of yoga stimulates and activates all the glands, organs, tissues and cells of the body. Yoga allows fresh, oxygenated blood flow to glands in the endocrine system to help relieve perimenopause symptoms.

Acupuncture is a proven treatment for hot flashes, joint pain, insomnia, and mood swings.

Menopause marks the end of menstruation and the average age is around 50. Conventional medicine view's menopause as a disease that needs to be treated. When in fact menopause is a natural transitional process. Conventional medical treatment of menopause is hormone replacement therapy that has significant risks and side effects. The natural treatment of menopause aims to balance hormone levels and encourage optimum health so your body can manage the natural transition with ease.

In Post menopause your hormone levels out and most of your symptoms disappeared. For many women, the years after menopause can be a very liberating time in their lives.

My Favorite Things

Favorite Things

These are some of my favorite products, recipes, and brands.

- Aubrey skin and hair care and cosmetics
  http://www.aubrey-organics.com/Affiliate.aspx?id=2808

- Giovanni Cosmetics — I love their shampoo.

- Ultra Aesthetics--This face care line is my absolute favorite! I have used it for years!

- Burt's Bees — A clean line, for the most part. Be sure to check the labels for ingredients to avoid. I love the color lip glosses!

- Dr. Bronner's Magic Soaps — I use the Peppermint and love it! It is a clean all purpose soap that moisturizes. It is wonderful for bathing dogs (it is all I use for my dogs and their hair is shiny, soft and healthy looking.

- Juicing first thing in the morning (my favorite is carrot, celery, beet)

- Veggie Broth — homemade so you can make in large quantities and freeze some to last longer! This way, you get a good dose of veggies every day! The pulp is great for disguising in cooked food for kids so they eat

veggies and do not even know it—
you will be surprised how much
better foods and even deserts taste
with the minced pulp added! Who
knew? It has fooled *my* family! You
just have to try this!

- My favorite detox herbal (dry herbs
  that you steep) are: Eyebright for
  blood cleansing, Red Clover for
  hormone balancing, and Peppermint
  for stomach and digestion

- Braggs Seasonings
Braggs All Purpose Seasoning is a salt
substitute that my entire family loves.
Braggs contains all eight essential amino
acids and is free of cholesterol and uric
acid. Braggs is made of soybeans and

water. Soybeans are converted into a liquid vegetable protein with no additives, preservatives, chemicals, coloring agents, or added sodium, and are easily digestible. Best of all, it tastes great!

Braggs contains the following essential and nonessential amino acids in naturally occurring amounts:

Alanine

Lysine

Valine

Arginine

Leucine

Aspartic Acid

Methioine

Glutamic Acid

Phenylalaine

Glycine

Proline

Histidine

Serine

Isoleucine

Threonine

Lysine Tyrosine

Where to find some of my favorites:

- Detox Foot Pads

  http://www.globalhealingcenter.com/af/173002

- Raw Food:

 http://www.1shoppingcart.com/app/?af=1142894

- Naturoli – A great site! Check it out!

- Himalayan Mineral

- Gurmukh Kundalini Yoga:

- Greens Plus Chocolate Energy Bar: It is Great Tasting! But even better it is chock full of living super-foods and High Energy Herbal Extracts. Just read the label to see all the wonderful ingredients in a delicious guilt free snack

Spirulina is a vegetable with more protein than soy, more Vitamin A than carrots, more iron than beef, and profound source of protective photochemical, naturally low in fat, source of essential fatty acids. Spirulina is available in powder form, as flakes, tablets, capsules or gel capsules. It is not the best tasting, so I only add very little of the powder to my herb tea or water. You cannot taste it them, but turns your water green so you know it is working.

- Roasted Seaweed is one of my favorite snacks. Seaweed is an excellent food because of its high nutritional values. Seaweed is low in Cholesterol and is a good source of vitamin B5 (beneficial for reducing cholesterol), Rheumatoid arthritis and Acne. Dried or roasted seaweed also contains Magnesium and Iron which are essential for preventing diabetes and heart attacks. Dried or roasted seaweed also contains Riboflavin and Niacin which promote fast tissue repair.

- Isenagix:
  http://drybarra.isagenix.com/us/en
  /landing_toxic.html

www.ingramcontent.com/pod-product-compliance
Lightning Source LLC
Chambersburg PA
CBHW070419290526
45791CB00005B/1756